Narcissism

How Narcissists Behave

What Causes Narcissism

What To Do About It

Cris Carter

First Printing, 2013

ISBN-13: 978-1492232117
ISBN-10: 1492232114

Printed in the United States of America

Disclaimer

This publication is designed to provide accurate and authoritative information in regard to the subject matter covered. It is sold with the understanding that the publisher is not engaged in rendering health, legal, counseling, or other professional services. If professional advice or other expert assistance is required, the services of a competent professional person should be sought. Designated trademarks and brands are the property of their respective owners.

DEDICATION

This book is dedicated to all of the health professionals and volunteers - physicians, nurses and research scientists and many more in the fight against mental illness.

CONTENTS

ACKNOWLEDGMENTS

I acknowledge and thank all those who made this book possible. My special thanks goes to Cynthia my Editor in Chief. Without your editing and input, this book would not be possible.

INTRODUCTION

Have you ever thought that someone in your life currently or someone you were involved with in the past is a narcissist? Perhaps you think that you may be living with one. You, or someone you know, could even have horrific stories to tell of Machiavellian encounters with your "loved one" that just wouldn't stop. You may think that you are being treated like an "object" used for their every desire or used like you are a slave and you just can't understand why.

Some poor souls who believe they have been victims of narcissism tell of going through hell, then ending up divorced and millions of dollars in debt. Or, you are positive your boss is a narcissist and you need to figure out how to deal with it or you are going to "go crazy" or resign before you do.

Maybe people have accused you of being a narcissist and you think this accusation is just a nasty way of telling you they think you are selfish. Of course, you are better than most everyone else. Why can't the world just accept it? Why won't everybody do what you tell them to do? They know you are always right! Or have you ever feared that because you have so many "broken" relationships that you are indeed a narcissist?

Narcissism is an often misunderstood and a misused term. There are many questions about it and some strong opinions about it as well. Here are some of the common comments and questions "heard on the street" about the hot topic of narcissism:

What is narcissism anyway? Is it really a mental problem that some people have or is it just a "bad personality type"? If it is a mental condition, how do you get it? Is it contagious? Is it "terminal"? Can it be treated with drugs? Why in the world would anybody call the love-of-self narcissistic? I heard that a certain amount of narcissism is healthy and without having it, you are going to get trampled on in life. Is this true? Where did this term come from?

Once you have narcissism, if it is real, can anybody really do anything about it? Can a doctor help my spouse or my boss or not? If so, what kind of doctor?

I may not be able to address every one of your questions about narcissism but by continuing to read on, you should get a good head start on the problem and perhaps be knowledgeable enough to know what to do next or at least know where to seek additional information.

1 WHAT IS NARCISSISM?

Where Did The Term Narcissism Come From?

The term is derived from Greek mythology about a Greek fellow named Narcissus who "gazed into a pool of water and fell in love with his own reflection". Supposedly, he was getting "hit on" by desperate nymphs and kept rejecting their advances. He decided to look into the pool to see what they were so attracted to. He began spending hours at the pool looking at his own reflection and then…turned into a flower. Do you know anybody like that? Would you like them to turn into a flower or, perhaps, something other than a flower?

The concept of narcissism as a mental disorder has slowly developed over the years. In the late 1800's the term, "narcissus-like", was used to describe people who "become their own sex object". Then in the early 1900's psychological papers began to pop up referring to narcissism as holding one's self with excessive high regard, admiration and showing signs of vanity. Sigmund Freud published a paper during this era as did Martin Buber using the term narcissism for people who do not relate to others as human beings normally do but view others and even "use" others more as objects.

Then starting around the turn of the century, the psychiatric community began to incorporate narcissism into the diagnosis and treatment of mental disorders. This is also when a set of psychological tests were beginning to be utilized as a standard practice in the diagnosis of the mental disorder formally named narcissism.

Many People Have and Still Do Question Whether Narcissism is A Real Mental Disorder

Many health professionals, researchers and the general public have asked the question: Is narcissism a clinical disorder? Some have, in the past, considered people who don't seem to care about others as merely possessing a self-centered personality. One that no one really wants to become friends with, much less live with, but it is not a "clinical disorder" that deserves any type of special medical treatment…surely not if insurance has to pay for it. There has even been an attitude out there about "healthy narcissism". Some have even espoused that being highly self-centered is really a good thing. If you don't "watch out for yourself", who is going to?

Is Narcissism A Real Mental Health Disorder?

Well, we can now put this kind of thinking to rest. All one has to do is refer to the DSM-5 which is the Diagnostic and Statistical Manual of Mental Disorders Version 5 published by the American Psychiatric Association. This is the manual that clinicians and physicians refer to when diagnosing mental disorders. Narcissism was officially declared a clinical disorder back in 1980 and there has been some official debate about whether it belongs in the manual or not. However, it remains there along with other personality disorders.

So the best way to define narcissism is the way the medical community does. Health professionals in the mental health community now define narcissism as a personality disorder. It is one of the five personality disorders listed in the DSM-5 and they are all classified as mental disorders.

In the DSM-5 there are five basic personality disorders. They are borderline, obsessive compulsive, schizotypal, antisocial, and narcissistic. According to the American Psychiatric Association each of these personality disorders has an explicit set of impaired personality behaviors and personality dysfunctions
.

However, clinicians can also diagnose what is known as PD-TS (personality disorder trait specified). This can be used when there is a personality disorder present as characterized by impaired and dysfunctional social behavior but the behavior does not meet the specific criteria of one of the disorders specified in the manual. When diagnosing narcissism the clinician or physician will look for specific personality traits and disorders specified as narcissistic traits.

2 DIAGNOSIS OF THE MENTAL DISORDER NARCISSISM

There is a narcissistic personality inventory (NPI) tool based on forced choice questions meant for measuring narcissism in populations of people and a diagnostic tool called the Millon Clinical Multiaxial Inventory (MCMI) used more for individual cases that can be and often are used by medical professionals to diagnose NPD (narcissist personality disorder). These tools can be helpful but they cannot be used by themselves. They must be used in conjunction with observations of patient behavior. In order to be diagnosed and get treatment for NPD, a patient's condition should meet the criteria for a diagnosis of NPD as defined in the Diagnostic and Statistical Manual of Mental Disorders (DSM-5).

NPD Behavioral Characteristics

The manifestations of narcissist personality disorder are an extreme (some even call it erotic) self-interest that often involves an emphasis on physical appearance. If one is diagnosed with narcissism personality disorder (NPD), it will generally result as a consequence of a psychiatrist or other qualified health professional observing the patient behaving as if he or she is without the capacity to love anyone but themselves. Most of the time they are unable to provide their significant other, friends and other family members with the love, friendship and caring they all need for a healthy two-way relationship.

Also, the patient exhibits a behavior totally lacking in empathy, disregarding other people's feelings and ignoring what others in their life care about. They have never "felt anyone else's pain" or even tried to empathize with someone going through a difficult time. In fact, there is only one perspective on the world that exists to the narcissist: their own.

With NPD the narcissist will often have an unrealistic and "out of touch with reality" overconfidence and vanity. They will view their appearance and capabilities as far better than they actually are yet they are unable to deal with even the slightest of criticism. They will hunger for and even demand praise and admiration from those in their life.

Other People Live To Meet The Needs Of The Narcissist

Relating to the early paper by Martin Buber referred to earlier in this book, Buber recognized that narcissists view other people as objects to be used for achieving their ends rather than treating people as equal human beings. They will use others to achieve their own ends without the slightest thought of what it may cost the other person

.

A Lack Of Appropriate Boundaries

This "people are objects to be used" attitude can create a very strange situation whereby the narcissist cannot distinguish between himself or herself and others. So the narcissistic views others as an extension of themselves and thinks that others exist only to meet their needs. If it turns out that the other people in their life do not exist for this purpose then the narcissist doesn't even recognize their existence.

That's right! Other people don't even exist in the mind of the narcissist if they are not living to meet the every need of the narcissist. This is called the lack of the ability to recognize boundaries. In other words, other people are extensions of themselves and are expected to behave the way the narcissist expects them to and live up to each and every one of their expectations. There is no boundary between the narcissist and others. For those that the narcissists view as true extensions of themselves, they heap on unwarranted flattery and admiration so as to maintain the affirmation of their unrealistic and inflated self worth.

Oblivious

Another behavior of the narcissist is a lack of awareness and insight. They have no idea they have a mental illness and are totally unaware of the impact their behavior has on others. This can make it very difficult to treat narcissists. This also makes it nearly impossible for them to have normal relationships with other people. All of their interaction with the other people in their lives is focused on themselves making the continuation of any kind of favorable two-way relation that they start extremely difficult for the other person.

Lack of Appropriate Emotion

The narcissist does not have the ability to feel appropriate relational emotions because their life is not about others…it's only about them. So not only do they not have normal love emotions, they also either repress totally or never really feel emotions like regret when they should. After hurting someone else emotionally, even committing acts of violence, when they should feel shame and remorse they do not. They live a life never apologizing, asking for forgiveness or for that matter even feeling bad about hurting other people emotionally or physically.

Conversely, when someone does something for them that is extraordinary and a person would normally feel the emotion of gratitude and thank them appropriately, the narcissist will not express gratitude. This is because everyone in the narcissist's life is expected to do wonderful things for the narcissist and it's not "normal" when they don't. In fact, as we will explore next, the emotion that is most likely felt when there is a lack of pandering and admiring the narcissist is called injury and rage.

Narcissist Injury and Rage

The fact that the narcissist cannot tolerate even the slightest criticism creates a cycle of never ending false injury then rage reaction to the perceived injury. Any interaction with someone that does not affirm the narcissists inflated ego is viewed as an insult and the narcissist feels emotionally injured. This "injury" most often is followed by a narcissist rage reaction. This reaction can be mild and take the form of an aloof demeanor, or an annoyed and irritated reaction, all the way to outbursts of anger. These episodes of anger can be quite frequent and can even lead to violent behavior. The anger is directed at, not only the perpetrators of the insults, but also inward toward himself or herself because the narcissist feels somehow that the narcissist did not live up to their impractical and "impossible to live up to" self-image. They will often end up detesting or even hating those that do not admire them and fit into their world where everyone lives only to please them.

3 OBSERVING NARCISSISTIC BEHAVIOR

Because of the ridiculous self-image the narcissist holds so dearly, they will exhibit certain characteristics inherent with the disorder. First of all, they will have a body language that can be called high and mighty, arrogant, conceited or snooty. They will also be unbelievably overconfident, lie about things they have accomplished that they have not accomplished and pretend to be more important than they obviously are.

All Of The Bragging Rights Belong To the Narcissist

They are braggarts to the extreme. Their bragging can be subtle and crafty so as not to be obvious and blatant about it, attempting to avoid getting caught in exaggerations. They can become very good at the "skill" of bragging. The bragging will be determined and unrelenting. If they do have provable achievements, they will always exaggerate the importance of the achievements they can prove. They will always act as if they are an expert at many things even if they do not know the slightest thing about the subject.

The Narcissist Is A Magical Thinker

At times the narcissist will display what you might call magical thinking about just how wonderful they are, what they know and what they can accomplish. They even will sometimes think that just because they believe something to be correct and true that it is in reality correct and true, even if there is strong evidence to the contrary. If it is obvious that the narcissist cannot "measure up" to someone else, they will often be envious and show disdain for and disapproval of the person to diminish them as much as possible.

The Entitled Narcissist

According to the narcissist he or she is entitled to get everything they want and are entitled to have every event in life go their way. They are entitled to the most favorable treatment wherever they go and everyone needs to comply with their wishes, their way of doing things and their way of thinking. They are always the special person in the relationship and not going along will classify the non complier as a difficult or dumb and awkward person in the narcissist's special world.

The Manipulating Narcissist

Often times other people will be forced into a subservient position by way of being an employee, spouse or child. Or sometimes the other person will just be timid and afraid to challenge the will and authority of the narcissist. The narcissist will start each new relationship assuming the other person is in a subservient position even when they are not. This puts the narcissist in a position of easily exploiting all who are unfortunate enough to find themselves in this position.

Narcissists of Many Colors

These behaviors and attitudes are what define the mental condition of the narcissist. The condition can assume varying degrees of severity. Some narcissists have such dysfunctional family and social relationships they end up alone, broken and unable to function in society. Others can master manipulation strategies and techniques so well that they become very successful in business or end up at the top of their very demanding professions finally accumulating an "entourage" of subordinates that take care of their every need, pander to their ego, swallow their pride and usually take their very substantial paychecks to the bank. However, narcissists usually fail at one thing in life. They fail at lasting relationships where love defines behavior because they only love themselves. They have a lifelong love affair with themselves "forever gazing into the pool at their own reflection".

Cris Carter

4 HEALTHY NARCISSISM

You can't begin to understand the personality disorder classified as NPD without investigating current thinking on so called "healthy narcissism". Everyone needs to feel good about themselves and pursue a life of achievement and success. It is very difficult, especially in our free market, competitive economy, to thrive in life if one carries the baggage of a negative self-image and goes through life without any self-confidence. This idea of healthy narcissism comes from a theory in psychology called object relations.

We All Are Objects In Someone's Subconscious

The idea is that adults will relate to others based on their experience as infants relating to their parents. Images of how they were treated as infants become "objects" in their subconscious. As adults, when other people remind them of their parents, the subconscious will predict how this person is going to behave toward them. If the object in their subconscious mind produces memories of mistreatment or neglect, or memories of happiness and nurturing, the behavior predicted by the subconscious will correspond to the memory. Thus the idea that people are treated as objects because of the objects that "live" in the subconscious formed in infancy and early childhood was "born" with this theory. The process of predicting at the subconscious level how someone is going to be treated by another has a tremendous effect on a person's family and social relationships.

A Healthy Relationship With Subconscious Objects And Therefore With Others In Life

A healthy narcissist will have subconscious objects that facilitate the proper behavior toward others they have relationships with, giving the healthy narcissist the ability to both receive and give gratifying engagements and have gratifying experiences with others in their life. Healthy subconscious objects help to build a truthful self-image that is in balance with the ego and there is no need to treat people as objects to be used solely for the purpose of achievement and self-aggrandizement.

The Causes Of Pathological Narcissism

It is reported that narcissism becomes unhealthy and pathological when one cannot love the objects stored in their subconscious and the frustration this creates produces an obsession with self-love and the megalomania behavior that follows.

5 DOING OUR BEST TO PREVENT NARCISSISM

Stay Away From Extreme Parenting

Look to the parents and/or primary caregivers of infants and young children to prevent or at least reduce the risk of narcissist personality disorder (NPD). Although there is some inconclusive research indicating that there may be hereditary and psychobiological factors that contribute to the disorder, the accepted thinking currently is that NPD is a result of how infants and young children are cared for. Because of the "macho male" culture we live in, males seem to be more susceptible to NPD than females; however, females also are at risk and can reach adulthood with NPD.

Teaching That It Is OK to Feel And Communicate Vulnerability At Appropriate Times

Parents that show disapproval of their children expressing fear or being needy are potentially creating conditions for narcissist tendencies to develop later in the child's life. Parents need to teach their children how to appropriately express their vulnerability to the right people at the right times for the right reasons and not suppress every fear or need they have.

Neglect and Abuse

Never showing affection, inflicting emotional and/or physical abuse or neglecting children are the worst parental sins for creating conditions prime for adult narcissism. These conditions can have devastating consequences.

Rewards and Praise

Also, rewarding and praising youngsters should be appropriate for the circumstance. Too much praise especially if it is not warranted, as well as indulging the child in bad behavior or a total lack of praise can all be damaging to a young and developing personality.

Can I Rely On Mom and Dad?

Another parenting mistake is allowing the care of the child to be inconsistent. The last thing, especially as infants, children need is to get the idea that their parents or primary caregivers are unreliable and possibly not there when needed and called for. The child needs to be able to predict with some certainty that their needs are going to be met within a reasonable period of time.

The Machiavellian Parent

Lastly, it seems that some of the best narcissist manipulators learn their manipulation skills from their parents. If parents are in the habit of getting what they want from their children with manipulative maneuvers, they are likely passing these "skills" on to their children and setting themselves up for a future of being manipulated by their children in addition to exposing others in the child's life such as teachers, their eventual spouse, coworkers and even the child's children to the same manipulative behavior.

Other Complicating Factors Driving NPD

There are other situational occurrences in a person's life that can "push someone over the edge into full blown NPD" if they are a borderline narcissist. Some of these situations will not surprise you such as alcohol or drug abuse. However, the risk can increase with other mental disorders such as depression especially when the condition is severe enough to cause suicidal thinking or attempts at suicide. Even normal life challenges such as close relationships that get into trouble or problems at work or school can trigger narcissist behaviors.

6 TREATMENT

Unless there are other mental disorders present such as depression or anxiety, it is not appropriate to treat narcissism with prescription medications. The disorder is treated with psychotherapy. However, it is important to treat other mental disorders if they are present with tranquilizers or antidepressant medication. These other mental problems need to be addressed or the patient may not respond favorably to psychotherapy methods. The goal of the treatment is to detect and reduce, if not eliminate altogether, dysfunctional thinking, beliefs and behavior, then gradually build up healthy ones to replace them.

Family and Group Therapy

This process may involve family or group therapy sessions because they are the foundation of relationships and in many cases the best place for healing to begin. After all, aren't relationship problems what NPD is about? Learning to have healthy relationships must involve and include other people. One of the benefits of family involvement if there are children involved is the possibility of breaking the cycle and doing everything possible so as not to pass the problem on to future generations.

The process, if it does work, may take several years and could require some tough lifestyle changes. An "all about me lifestyle" cannot continue.

8 CONCLUSION

As you can see, narcissism can be a complicated and difficult to live with mental disorder. Know however that NPD, narcissist personality disorder, is a "real" mental health disorder and the manifestations and dysfunctional behaviors associated with it should not be dismissed as just having a selfish personality.

The pain and suffering inflicted by the narcissist can be punishing and severe. There can be plenty of pain to go around as the narcissist manipulates his or her spouse, coworkers and everyone else to whatever end the narcissist has in mind. The lack of love, empathy, sympathy, compassion, shame and remorse is devastating to the family and prevents the narcissist from ever having any long-lasting, healthy relationships with anyone.

It can exist without any other mental health disorders or with them. If you suspect that someone you care about has this disorder, you should encourage them to seek professional treatment. If they will not, which is often the case as they usually deny that anything is wrong with them, you need to do whatever is necessary to protect yourself and the well being of your family.

If you are the one struggling with this disorder, the best thing you can do is seek assistance from qualified professionals trained to help with these and other serious mental disorders. Start with your family physician and get a referral for the best care you can seek. There is hope and help.

Lastly, be vigilant and please don't practice extreme parenting. Your children deserve better!